Rucking for Healthy Aging and Weight Loss After 50

A Safe, Low-Impact Way to Stay Fit for Life

Chuck Finley

Table of Contents

Introduction: Why Walk When You Can Ruck?   01

- The case for rucking after 50
- Why "simple" beats "complicated" fitness
- What this book will give you

Chapter 1: Why Rucking? The Perfect Fitness Tool After 50   04

- The Fitness Industry's Dirty Little Secret
- Walking With Purpose (and a Backpack)
- Why It Works After 50
- Busting the Biggest Myths
- Tina's Story
- The Bottom Line

Chapter 2: Preparing Your Body and Mind   10

- Setting Realistic Goals (AKA Don't Try to Become Rambo Overnight)
- Mindset for Success
- Assessing Your Starting Point
- Safety First (Because Pulling a Hamstring Is Not a Fitness Goal)
- The Bottom Line

Chapter 3: Gear Up — Equipment Made Simple   16

- Choosing the Right Backpack (Your New Best Friend)
- Weight Selection (Less Is More…At First)
- Footwear Matters (Because Blisters Are Not a Badge of Honor)
- Clothing and Accessories (Keep It Simple, Keep It Smart)
- The Bottom Line

Chapter 4: Building Your Rucking Foundation 22

- Starting Small (Rome Wasn't Built in a Day)
- Proper Rucking Technique (How to Walk Like a Pro)
- Structuring Your Routine (Consistency Beats Intensity)
- Monitoring Progress (Celebrate the Small Wins)
- Your 12-Week Beginner Rucking Plan
- The Bottom Line

Chapter 5: Advancing Your Rucking Practice 22

- Increasing Intensity Safely (Level Up Without Falling Apart)
- Adding Variety (Because Boredom Is the Real Enemy)
- Overcoming Plateaus (When Progress Stalls)
- Integrating Rucking into Daily Life (The Sneaky Fitness Hack)
- Your 12-Week Advanced Rucking Plan
- The Bottom Line

Chapter 6: Rucking for Life — Long-Term Health and Motivation 43

Weight Loss and Healthy Aging (Why Rucking Works When Diets Don't)
Lifelong Fitness and Mobility (Staying Independent and Strong)
Building a Community (Because Everything's Better Together)
Your Next Steps (Turning Rucking Into a Lifestyle)
The Bottom Line

Epilogue: Ruck Up and Step Forward 49

The secret formula in one line
Why the first step matters most
The lifelong challenge

INTRODUCTION: WHY WALK WHEN YOU CAN RUCK?

Let's face it—you're not here because life after 50 has been all six-pack abs, endless energy, and a metabolism that lets you eat pizza at midnight without consequences. No, you're here because something's changed. Maybe it's the stubborn weight that laughs at your old tricks. Maybe it's the joints that creak like a haunted house when you climb stairs. Or maybe it's the simple realization that if you don't take charge now, you might spend your so-called "golden years" sitting on the sidelines instead of living fully.

But I've got good news: the solution doesn't require a CrossFit membership, a second mortgage for fancy fitness gear, or becoming that person who orders kale at every meal. Instead, it's something almost insultingly simple: put on a backpack, add some weight, and go for a walk. That's it. Congratulations, you've discovered rucking.

Now, before you roll your eyes and say, "Really? Walking with a bag is supposed to change my life?"—hear me out. Rucking is like fitness's best-kept secret.

It burns more calories than regular walking, builds strength without wrecking your knees, and has been used for centuries by soldiers, athletes, and, yes, regular people who want to look and feel better.

It's also ridiculously beginner-friendly. If you can walk, you can ruck. If you can't walk...well, start by reading this book, and we'll get you moving in the right direction.

Think of rucking as the middle ground between strolling through the park and running a marathon. You don't need to be an athlete. You don't need to be "in shape." You don't even need to enjoy exercise (though don't worry—you might actually learn to like this). What you do need is the willingness to try something new, something effective, and something that just might become the most enjoyable part of your week.

This book will take you from "What the heck is rucking?" to "Why didn't I start this years ago?" Along the way, we'll talk about how to set goals you'll actually stick to, the gear you need (spoiler: not much), how to stay safe, and how to make rucking a habit that supports healthy aging, weight loss, and—let's not forget—having fun.

By the time you finish, you'll not only know how to start rucking, you'll be itching to lace up your shoes, throw some weight on your back, and hit the road. And here's the kicker: you'll realize that you don't need to slow down with age—you just need the right strategy to keep going strong.

So, if you're ready to laugh at the idea of "over the hill," trade sluggishness for strength, and maybe even surprise your friends when they ask, "Wait—you've been doing what with a backpack?" ... then let's get started.

CHAPTER 1
WHY RUCKING?
The Perfect Fitness Tool After 50

The Fitness Industry's Dirty Little Secret

Let's get real: the fitness industry thrives on making people believe that exercise has to be complicated, expensive, and ideally purchased in 12 easy installments of $39.99. One week it's high-intensity spin classes, the next it's goat yoga, and the week after that it's some influencer selling resistance bands that look suspiciously like the bungee cords in your garage.

But here's the secret most gyms and gadget companies don't want you to know: you don't need any of that to get fit, lose weight, or age gracefully. What you actually need is a sustainable, effective, low-impact form of movement that builds strength and burns calories without destroying your joints.

Enter rucking.

Rucking is so simple that it almost feels like cheating. You take walking—a basic human activity you've been doing since you were a toddler—and you add a backpack with some weight. That's it. No subscriptions. No complicated workout charts. No Lycra bodysuits required (unless you're into that sort of thing, in which case, rock on).

Walking With Purpose (and a Backpack)

Here's the truth: walking is already a powerhouse for your health. Study after study shows that people who walk regularly live longer, maintain healthier weights, and keep their brains sharper. Walking is like the Swiss Army knife of exercise—it's good for just about everything.

But rucking takes that Swiss Army knife and straps a chainsaw to it. By adding even a modest amount of weight to your walk, you transform a leisurely stroll into a workout that makes your heart pump harder, your muscles work overtime, and your calorie burn skyrocket.

Think about it: carrying groceries up the stairs, lugging a suitcase through an airport, or hauling a grandkid on your back—these are all real-life forms of rucking.

Why It Works After 50

Aging comes with some unavoidable realities. Metabolism slows down. Muscle mass declines. Bones weaken. And sometimes, your knees remind you they've been around the block a few too many times. The typical advice is to either:

1. Start running (hello, knee pain!)
2. Lift heavy weights (intimidating and not always safe without guidance)
3. Or just...accept decline as "part of aging."

Yeah, no thanks.

Rucking is the Goldilocks solution: not too hard, not too easy, and just right for keeping your body strong without punishing it.

- **It builds strength and endurance simultaneously.** Every step with weight strengthens your legs, back, and core while giving your heart a workout.

- **It's joint-friendly.** Unlike running, rucking doesn't hammer your knees, hips, or ankles into submission.

- **It's scalable.** Start with 10 pounds for 10 minutes. Over time, increase weight, distance, or pace. You're in control of the progression.

Best of all, it fits seamlessly into your life. No rearranging your schedule to hit the gym. No weird choreography to memorize. Just grab your pack, step outside, and go.

Busting the Biggest Myths

Before you start, let's clear up a few misconceptions that might be floating around in your head:

- **"I'm too old to carry weight."** Actually, carrying weight is exactly what you should be doing—safely, of course. It strengthens bones, muscles, and connective tissues, which is crucial for preventing falls and injuries later in life. Think of it as future-proofing your body.

- **"Walking isn't real exercise."** Tell that to your heart rate after a 30-minute ruck. The beauty of rucking is that it feels deceptively easy, but your body knows it's working. And unlike "beast mode" workouts, you won't be lying on the floor questioning your life choices afterward.

- **"I need fancy equipment."** Nope. If you own a backpack and have access to heavy objects (books, water bottles, canned soup, etc.), you already have everything you need to start. Don't let the social media ads convince you otherwise.

Tina

Real quick, I need to mention Tina. My neighbors often see me walking around with my rucksack. Early one morning, I ran into Tina. She was out walking her dog, she introduced herself and Bowzer, and she mentioned that she sees me frequently out with my backpack on. I, with much enthusiasm, explained my workout to her and how easy it is to get started. Tina was interested, but her biggest concern was the cost. I asked her, "do you have an old backpack"? She was sure there had to be one or two house somewhere. We talked about starting out slowly, that there was no need for expensive weights in the backpack, and Tina seemed genuinely excited about the idea.

Fast forward about 2 weeks, and I ran into her again. Tina, who I should mention is slightly younger than me, was proudly showing me the backpack she found, and explaining how she filled little paper bags with exactly one pound of stones each. She currently had six bags in her backpack, and her mom, who was walking with Tina and also wearing a backpack, had four in hers. I grinned all the way home.

Start with what you have. The hardest part isn't the weight—it's the first step.

The Bottom Line

Rucking is the ultimate fitness hack after 50: it's simple, scalable, safe, and ridiculously effective. It's exercise disguised as something anyone can do, which is why it works so well. You don't need to run marathons, deadlift your bodyweight, or become a yoga pretzel to age well—you just need to walk with purpose and a little extra weight.

The beauty of rucking is that it puts you back in the driver's seat. You're not just slowing the effects of aging—you're actively fighting them. And while your peers might complain about slowing down, you'll be getting stronger, leaner, and healthier with every step.

So, now that you know why rucking deserves a spot in your life, the next step is to prepare your body and mind for the journey. In the next chapter, we'll talk about setting realistic goals, building confidence, and making sure your body is ready to start this new adventure.

And don't worry—we'll leave kale smoothies out of it.

CHAPTER 2

PREPARING YOUR BODY AND MIND

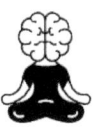

Setting Realistic Goals (AKA: Don't Try to Become Rambo Overnight)

One of the biggest mistakes people make when starting a new fitness routine is going in like they're auditioning for an action movie. They buy all the gear, load up their bag with 50 pounds, and set off like they're invading Normandy—only to come back limping, swearing, and vowing never to do it again.

That's not the plan here. You don't need to become Rambo. You just need to become a slightly fitter, healthier version of you.

Start by asking yourself: *What do I want from this?* If your goal is weight loss, rucking will help.

If your goal is aging gracefully while still being able to pick up your grandkids or your groceries without grunting like a powerlifter—rucking's got you covered. If your goal is training for your secret dream of joining the Army Rangers at 55...well, I admire your ambition, but let's walk before we ruck-march.

Pro tip: Set goals you can actually achieve. For example:

- "I'll ruck twice a week for 20 minutes." (Doable.)

- "I'll lose 10 pounds in two weeks by rucking every day and eating only lettuce." (Please don't.)

Mindset for Success

Here's the truth: motivation is overrated. Sure, it feels great when you're fired up, but motivation is like that flaky friend who shows up late—if at all. What you actually need is consistency. And consistency comes from mindset.

Think of rucking not as "exercise" but as "maintenance." Like brushing your teeth, mowing the lawn, or making coffee every morning—it's just something you *do*.

A beginner's mindset will carry you far. Don't worry if you're slow.

Don't stress if your backpack looks more like a school kid's lunchbox than a tactical military ruck. Every step you take with weight is a win. You're training your body, rewiring your brain, and telling Father Time he can shove it.

Here's how to build the right mindset:

1. **Lower the barrier to entry.** Promise yourself just 10 minutes. Once you're out the door, you'll usually do more.

2. **Detach from "all-or-nothing" thinking.** Missing a day isn't failure; it's life. Just pick it back up.

3. **Remember your "why."** You're not just walking with a bag—you're investing in years of future strength, independence, and vitality.

Assessing Your Starting Point

Before you strap on a pack and head out like a weekend warrior, let's do a quick reality check. No shame, no judgment—just a clear-eyed look at where you're starting.

- **Fitness self-assessment:** Can you walk comfortably for 15–20 minutes without pain? Can you carry a grocery bag without needing a nap afterward? Good. You're ready.

- **Doctor check-in:** If you've got existing health issues (blood pressure, heart concerns, joint problems), it's smart to get medical clearance. Think of your doctor as your rucking pit crew—they'll help you keep the engine running smoothly.

- **Listen to your body:** A little muscle soreness is fine. Sharp pain? Not fine. Breathing harder than usual is normal. Seeing stars and feeling dizzy? Not normal. Learn the difference, and don't ignore red flags.

The point isn't to pass some fitness test. The point is to start safely and build from there. If your starting point is slow and light, so what? You're still ahead of everyone sitting on the couch. Ruck Yeah!

Safety First (Because Pulling a Hamstring Is Not a Fitness Goal)

I know—safety sounds boring. But nothing derails fitness faster than an injury, and the good news is that with rucking, injuries are mostly preventable if you follow a few basics.

- **Warm up, don't just take off.** Think of your muscles like old rubber bands—give them a little stretch and movement before you load them up. A brisk 5-minute walk before adding your pack works wonders.

- **Cool down afterward.** A couple minutes of light stretching or walking without weight helps your body recover. Bonus points if you do some gentle hip and hamstring stretches.

- **Know the difference between pain and discomfort.** Rucking will make your muscles burn a little—that's good. Stabbing pain in your knees or back? That's your body saying "stop, genius."

- **Build gradually.** Don't let your ego talk you into throwing 40 pounds in your pack on day one. Progress is about patience, not punishment.

Think of safety as insurance: it's the boring stuff that protects the fun stuff. By being smart upfront, you'll ensure you get the long-term benefits without the setbacks.

The Bottom Line

Preparing your body and mind is the secret sauce of successful rucking. This isn't about going hard, fast, or heavy right away—it's about setting yourself up for consistent, enjoyable progress.

By setting realistic goals, adopting the right mindset, checking your starting point, and respecting safety, you're giving yourself the foundation to turn rucking from "just another workout" into a lifestyle.

Because here's the truth: fitness after 50 isn't about chasing perfection. It's about building resilience, staying active, and keeping your quality of life high. And rucking is one of the simplest, most effective ways to do exactly that.

Next up: Gear Up—Equipment Made Simple. Don't worry, this isn't an excuse to spend your retirement savings on tactical camo backpacks and titanium water bottles. We'll break down what you actually need (and what you can skip) so you can get started without draining your

CHAPTER 3

GEAR UP — EQUIPMENT MADE SIMPLE

Choosing the Right Backpack (Your New Best Friend)

Let's clear this up right away: you do not need a $300 "tactical" rucksack that looks like it's designed for surviving the zombie apocalypse. Unless you actually plan on fighting zombies (in which case, respect).

For beginners, the best ruck is the one you already own. Got an old school backpack? Perfect. Something your kids left behind after high school? Even better—free is the right price. The point is comfort, not combat readiness.

I can't stress that point enough, use what you have! I have little doubt that you will quickly come to love rucking as I have, but it will feel even better when you haven't invested a lot of money. When you get to that point where you are constantly looking forward to your next journey, maybe then it will be time to reward yourself with an upgraded ruck!

What to look for:

- **Durability.** You want something that won't rip the first time you load it with books. (Retirement funds don't need to go toward duct tape.)

- **Comfort.** Wide shoulder straps beat thin ones. Bonus points if there's a padded back.

- **Size.** Big enough to carry some weight but not so big you could smuggle a small llama inside.

If you stick with rucking and decide you love it, sure—upgrade to a sturdier pack. But don't let gear be an excuse to delay starting. Remember: it's not the bag that makes you fit; it's the steps you take with it.

Weight Selection (Less Is More...At First)

Here's where a lot of eager rookies mess up. They think, "If 10 pounds is good, 40 pounds must be amazing!" That's like saying, "If one cookie is tasty, eating the whole box is the best idea ever." Spoiler: it's not.

Start light. Ten to fifteen pounds is plenty to begin with. You'll be shocked at how different walking feels with even that small amount. Once you're comfortable, you can gradually add more weight over time.

Easy starter weights:

- Books (finally, your old encyclopedia set has a use).
- Gallons of water (8 pounds each).
- Dumbbells or weight plates (if you have them lying around).

Pro tip: Wrap your weights in a towel or pillowcase so they don't jab you in the back mid-walk. Unless you enjoy the feeling of being stabbed by *War and Peace*.

The goal isn't to punish yourself—it's to challenge yourself just enough to make progress. Think "gentle nudge," not "backyard Navy SEAL training camp."

Footwear Matters (Because Blisters Are Not a Badge of Honor)

You wouldn't run a marathon in flip-flops (I hope), and you shouldn't ruck in shoes that don't support your feet. Your feet are the MVPs of this whole operation—take care of them.

Here's the breakdown:

- **Walking shoes:** Great if you're sticking to sidewalks or smooth trails.

- **Hiking shoes/boots:** Better for uneven terrain. Bonus ankle support.

- **Running shoes:** Can work if they're supportive, but beware of flimsy soles.

And let's not forget socks. Good socks are like good friends: they protect you, support you, and don't leave you with blisters at the end of the day. Look for moisture-wicking socks made of synthetic blends or wool (yes, wool—even in summer, they keep your feet dry).

Invest here before you invest in a fancy ruck. Because let me tell you, nothing ends a new fitness habit faster than a blister the size of a silver dollar.

Clothing and Accessories (Keep It Simple, Keep It Smart)

Forget the idea that you need to look like a catalog model on your rucks. Rucking isn't a fashion show—it's functional fitness. That said, a little smart planning goes a long way.

Clothing:

- Weather-appropriate. Shorts and a T-shirt in summer, layers in winter.

- Moisture-wicking. Cotton holds sweat and chafes. Synthetic or wool is better.

- Comfort first. If it pinches, rubs, or annoys you standing still, it'll be 100x worse after 20 minutes.

Accessories:

- **Water bottle or hydration bladder.** Yes, even short rucks. Dehydrated zombies are not cool.

- **Reflective vest or lights.** If you're out at night, be seen. Nobody wants their workout cut short by a distracted driver.

- Headlamp. If you're an early bird or night owl, light your path. Falling into a ditch is not the kind of "intensity" we're going for.

- Optional bonus gear: a hat (for sun), sunglasses (for style and sun), and maybe a watch or app to track distance. But again—don't get paralyzed by shopping lists. The best accessory is just showing up.

The Bottom Line

Getting started with rucking doesn't require a shopping spree! All you need is a backpack, some weight, shoes that won't murder your feet, and clothes that keep you comfortable.

Don't let gear become a barrier. Fancy backpacks won't make you healthier—*rucking* will. Start with what you've got, improve as you go, and remember: the only truly essential piece of equipment is your commitment.

Now that you've got your gear sorted, it's time to put it to use. In the next chapter, we'll talk about **Building Your Rucking Foundation**—how to start small, master your technique, and create a routine that will actually stick. Because showing up is half the battle, but showing up smart is how you win the war.

CHAPTER 4

BUILDING YOUR RUCKING FOUNDATION

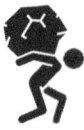

Starting Small (Because Rome Wasn't Built in a Day... And Neither Was Your Endurance)

If you've ever tried starting a fitness routine by going all-in from day one, you already know how that ends: sore muscles, cranky joints, and a sudden urge to never do that again. That's not our plan here.

We're building a foundation, and foundations are laid brick by brick—not by dropping a concrete slab on your head. Start with short, light rucks. Ten to twenty minutes with a light load (think 10–15 pounds) is more than enough. Trust me, you'll feel it.

Why start small?

- It builds confidence. Success creates momentum.

- It conditions your body safely. Your muscles, joints, and bones adapt without rebellion.

- It keeps you coming back. Nobody quits something that feels manageable and—even better—enjoyable.

Your first rucks aren't about "beast mode." They're about creating a habit. That backpack is your gateway drug to long-term fitness, not a medieval torture device.

Proper Rucking Technique (How to Walk Like a Pro)

You might be thinking, *"It's walking, how complicated can it be?"* Fair question. But just like lifting weights, a little technique goes a long way in preventing injury and maximizing results.

- **Posture matters.** Stand tall, shoulders back, chest open. Don't hunch forward like you're sneaking Halloween candy.

- **Stride naturally.** No stomping, no shuffling. Walk how you normally walk—just more aware of your steps.

- **Engage your core.** Think "tight but not tense." A braced core protects your spine and helps carry the load.

- **Breathe rhythmically.** Inhale for two steps, exhale for two steps. This keeps you from gasping like a fish halfway through.

- **Watch where you're going.** Especially on those neglected sidewalks, pay attention. Tripping and falling can hurt, tripping and falling with an additional 10-15 pounds on your back hurts a little more.

Pro tip: Imagine you're walking like someone confident and strong—because that's exactly what you're becoming.

Structuring Your Routine (Consistency Beats Intensity)

Now that you've taken your first rucks, let's put some structure behind them. Remember: the goal is progress you can stick with, not a one-week fling that ends in sore regret.

Beginner schedule idea:

- **2–3 times per week.** Start with non-consecutive days to allow recovery.//
- **10–20 minutes per ruck.** Keep it short and sweet.
- **10–15 pounds. Enough to feel it, but not enough to regret it.**

As weeks go by, you can *increase either* the distance or the weight—but not both at once. (Your joints will thank you.) Aim for slow, steady progress, not social media glory shots.

Think of this routine as your "base camp." You'll build from here, but you don't climb Everest on day one.

Monitoring Progress (Celebrate the Small Wins)

Progress tracking isn't about spreadsheets or military-grade data analysis. It's about giving yourself proof that you're moving forward—literally and figuratively.

Easy ways to track:

- **Distance.** Use a phone app, a watch, or even old-school pen and paper.

- **Time.** Write down how long you walked.

- **Weight carried.** Note how much you had in your pack.

And here's the fun part: celebrate the little victories. Walked five minutes longer than last time? That's a win. Carried an extra five pounds without collapsing? Another win. Completed three rucks in a week? You're crushing it.

Too often, people get caught up in what they *can't* do yet. Flip that script. Focus on what you're accomplishing, and let those small wins fuel your next steps.

Your 12-Week Beginner Rucking Plan

Alright, it's time to move from "thinking about rucking" to actually *doing* it. To help, here's a simple, progressive 12-week plan designed for anyone over 50 who wants to build endurance, strength, and confidence without wrecking their joints.

The rules of the road:

- **Ruck 3x per week** on non-consecutive days (e.g., Mon/Wed/Sat).

- **Start light.** Use 10–15 lbs. in a backpack. (Water bottles, books, or a dumbbell wrapped in a towel work great.)

- **Progress gradually.** You'll add either distance or weight, but never both in the same week.

- **Listen to your body.** If something feels wrong, scale back. The goal is longevity, not punishment.

Weeks 1–4: Building the Habit

- **Goal:** Get comfortable with the basics.

- **Load:** 10–15 lbs.

- **Sessions:** 3 per week.

Week	Duration Per Ruck	Notes
1	15 min	Focus on posture & breathing.
2	20 min	Keep same weight, just add time
3	25 min	Celebrate your first "long" ruck!
4	30 min	Stay steady—don't rush.

Weeks 5–8: Adding Distance & Challenge

- **Goal**: Increase endurance safely.

- **Load:** 15–20 lbs. (add 5 lbs. if comfortable).

- **Sessions:** 3 per week.

Week	Duration Per Ruck	Notes
5	30 min	Add light hills if available.
6	35 min	Keep steady pace. Hydrate well.
7	40 min	Take one ruck outdoors on varied terrain.
8	45 min	You're officially in "fitness routine" territory.

Weeks 9–12: Strength & Stamina Gains

- **Goal:** Build capacity and confidence.

- **Load:** 20–25 lbs. (gradually, as tolerated).

- **Sessions:** 3 per week.

Week	Duration Per Ruck	Notes
9	45 min	Add weight, not speed.
10	50 min	Try brisk pace for last 5–10 minutes.
11	55 min	Mix in short intervals: 2 min brisk / 3 min easy.
12	60 min	Victory lap—1 full hour with your pack!

Bonus Options (If You're Feeling Spicy)

- **The Grocery Grab:** Take your pack to the store, load it with groceries, and walk home (built-in strength training).

- **The Social Ruck:** Invite a friend or family member. Talking while rucking makes time fly and boosts accountability. It's working well for Tina and her mom!

- **The Scenic Route:** Find a park, trail, or waterfront. Fresh air and scenery make workouts feel less like work.

The Bottom Line

Building your rucking foundation isn't about speed, strength, or distance—it's about creating consistency. By starting small, focusing on technique, structuring your routine, and celebrating progress, you're setting yourself up for long-term success.

Remember: the only bad ruck is the one you didn't take. Every step with weight is a deposit in your future health account, and the returns compound faster than any retirement plan.

This 12-week plan isn't just about getting fitter—it's about proving to yourself that you can build strength, endurance, and resilience at any age. By the end, you'll be walking longer, carrying more, and feeling stronger than you thought possible. And the best part? You'll be ready to take your rucking to the next level.

Next chapter, we'll talk about **Advancing Your Rucking Practice**—because once you've built this foundation, it's time to have some fun with hills, intervals, and other ways to keep improving without getting bored.

CHAPTER 5

ADVANCING YOUR RUCKING PRACTICE

Increasing Intensity Safely (How to Level Up Without Falling Apart)

By now, you've built your foundation. You can ruck for 30–60 minutes, carry 15–25 pounds without needing an ice bath, and you've probably noticed your clothes fitting better (bonus points if someone's asked, "Have you been working out?").

Now it's time to make things more interesting. But here's the golden rule: **increase gradually**. Progress in rucking is like seasoning chili—you add a little bit at a time. Dump in the whole spice rack, and you'll regret it.

Here are safe ways to turn up the dial:

- **Add distance first.** Go from 2 miles to 2.5, then 3. Your body adapts naturally to more time on your feet.

- **Then add weight.** Once you're comfy at a distance, bump your load by 5 pounds. (Think of it as upgrading from "carry-on bag" to "checked luggage.")

- **Play with pace.** A brisker pace burns more calories and builds cardiovascular fitness. No need to jog—just walk like you're late to catch a plane.

Rule of thumb: change only one variable (distance, weight, or pace) at a time. Your joints and muscles will thank you.

Adding Variety (Because Boredom Is the Real Enemy)

Let's face it: walking the same route at the same pace, week after week, gets about as exciting as watching paint dry. The solution? Mix it up. Variety not only keeps your brain engaged, but it also challenges your body in new ways.

Here are a few ideas:

- **Hills.** Nature's stairmaster. Walking uphill with a ruck cranks up intensity and builds serious leg strength.

- **Terrain changes.** Swap the sidewalk for trails, grass, or sand. Your stabilizer muscles will get a workout.

- **Group rucks.** Everything's easier (and more fun) with company. Plus, you'll push yourself more without even noticing.

Pro tip: treat rucking like an adventure, not a chore. Try new neighborhoods, parks, or hiking trails. Think of it as fitness tourism.

Overcoming Plateaus (AKA: What to Do When Progress Stalls)

No matter how motivated you are, at some point your progress will slow down. You'll carry the same weight, walk the same distance, and think, *"Why am I not improving?"* Don't panic—it's normal.

Here's how to break through:

1. Change one variable. If you've been rucking 3 miles with 20 pounds forever, try 3.5 miles. Or keep the distance but add 5 pounds.

Remember: progress isn't always linear. Some weeks you'll crush it. Others you'll feel sluggish. What matters is sticking with the process.

Integrating Rucking into Daily Life (The Sneaky Fitness Hack)

Here's where rucking shines compared to most workouts: it's not just exercise—it's practical. You can weave it into your life without rearranging your schedule.

Ideas for sneaky integration:

- **Errands.** Strap on your ruck for a walk to the store, post office, or even your kid's soccer practice.

- **Social time.** Instead of coffee dates, suggest a "walk and talk" ruck. (Bonus: you'll burn calories while solving the world's problems.)

- **Commuting.** Live within a few miles of work, church, or a friend's house? That's a built-in ruck opportunity.

The more you blend rucking into everyday life, the less it feels like "exercise" and the more it becomes simply...*living better.*

Your 12-Week Advanced Rucking Plan

So you've finished the beginner plan, and you're feeling good—stronger, leaner, and maybe even a little smug when you zip past younger folks on the trail. Congrats! You've built the foundation. Now it's time to level up.

This 12-week advanced program introduces more distance, more weight, and some spicy variety (hills, intervals, and faster paces) to keep the gains rolling.

The rules of the road:

- **Ruck 3–4x per week.** Non-consecutive days if possible.

- **Alternate focus.** Some rucks focus on distance, others on speed, others on strength (weight).

- **Progress smartly.** Don't add distance *and* weight in the same week.

- **Deload if needed.** If you feel beat up, repeat the previous week before moving forward.

Weeks 1–4: Strengthening the Base

- **Goal:** Adapt to heavier loads while maintaining good form.

- **Load:** 20–25 lbs.

- **Sessions:** 3x/week (2 distance, 1 brisk).

Week	Distance Per Ruck	Focus
1	3 miles	Comfortable pace, focus on posture.
2	3.5 miles	Add a brisk pace day (walk like you're late).
3	4 miles	Include hills if possible.
4	4.5 miles	End one session with 5–10 minutes faster pace.

Weeks 5–8: Endurance & Variety

- **Goal:** Push endurance and introduce interval training.

- **Load:** 25–30 lbs.

- **Sessions:** 3x/week (2 distance, 1 interval).

Week	Distance Per Ruck	Focus
5	5 miles	2 steady, 1 interval (2 min brisk / 3 min easy).
6	5.5 miles	Add an optional 4th light ruck (3 miles, 15 lbs.).
7	6 miles	Keep interval session, add hills.
8	6.5 miles	Longest ruck this phase—pace yourself.

Weeks 9–12: Power & Pace

- **Goal:** Increase stamina and challenge speed under load.

- **Load:** 30–35 lbs.

- **Sessions:** 4x/week (2 distance, 1 brisk, 1 interval).

Week	Distance Per Ruck	Focus
9	5-6 miles	2 steady, 1 interval (2 min brisk / 3 min easy).
10	6-7 miles	Add an optional 4th light ruck (3 miles, 15 lbs.).
11	7 miles	Keep interval session, add hills.
12	8 miles	Longest ruck this phase—pace yourself.

Bonus Challenges (For the Truly Adventurous)

- **The Weighted Errand:** Ruck to the store, buy a bag of groceries, carry it home in your pack. (Functional fitness at its finest.)

- **The Charity Ruck:** Sign up for a local event—many rucking groups raise money for causes by doing long rucks together.

- **The Family Ruck:** Invite your spouse, kids, or grandkids. (Warning: you may get shown up by a 12-year-old, but hey, family bonding counts.)

The Bottom Line

Advancing your rucking practice doesn't mean turning it into a punishment. It means gently nudging yourself forward—more distance here, a little weight there, a hill climb to spice things up. Over time, these small changes add up to huge gains in strength, endurance, and confidence.

The best part? You'll never hit that "I'm too old for this" wall. Because rucking is infinitely adaptable—you scale it to your needs, your fitness, and your lifestyle.

The advanced 12-week plan is about proving to yourself that fitness after 50 isn't about slowing down—it's about scaling up. With heavier loads, longer distances, and a touch of variety, you'll not only keep your progress alive but also make rucking a long-term part of your lifestyle.

Remember: this isn't about suffering. It's about challenging yourself, one smart step at a time. And by the end of this plan, you won't just be "doing rucking." You'll *become a rucker (and if you're a mom, you're a mother-rucker...sorry, had to slip that in somewhere).*

Next, we'll wrap it all together in **Chapter 6: Rucking for Life—Long-Term Health and Motivation.** This is where you'll see how rucking supports weight loss, healthy aging, and, most importantly, staying strong and capable.

CHAPTER 6

RUCKING FOR LIFE — LONG-TERM HEALTH AND MOTIVATION

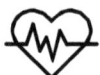

Weight Loss and Healthy Aging (Why Rucking Works When Diets Don't)

By now, you've probably noticed something: rucking feels different from other "exercise." You're not gasping on the floor like you just survived a boot camp class. You're not trying to remember the difference between a Romanian deadlift and a stiff-legged one. You're just...walking with weight. And yet the results sneak up on you.

Here's why:

- **Calorie burn.** Rucking torches more calories than regular walking. Without the joint-smashing impact of running, you can do more of it—consistently.

- **Metabolism booster.** Muscle is metabolically active tissue, and rucking helps you preserve (and even build) muscle. Translation: you burn more calories at rest.

- **Appetite control.** Unlike high-intensity workouts that leave you craving an entire pizza, rucking often suppresses appetite temporarily. Bonus: it makes healthy eating easier to stick to.

The real magic? Rucking isn't a crash-and-burn program. It's not "30 days to shredded abs." It's steady, sustainable, and effective—exactly what you need for long-term weight loss and aging like a boss.

Lifelong Fitness and Mobility (Staying Independent and Strong)

Here's the blunt truth: aging is optional, but decline isn't. If you do nothing, you'll lose muscle, bone density, balance, and independence. But if you ruck regularly, you stack the deck in your favor.

Rucking helps with:

- **Bone density.** Weight-bearing exercise is one of the best defenses against osteoporosis.

- **Balance and stability.** Walking with weight challenges your core and stabilizer muscles, helping you avoid falls.

- **Functional strength.** Want to pick up your grandkids? Carry luggage through the airport? Load a bag of mulch into your garden? Rucking trains you for *real life.*

Think of rucking as future-proofing your body. It's not about living forever—it's about living better for as long as you're here.

Building a Community (Because Everything's Better Together)

One of the underrated joys of rucking is that it doesn't have to be a solo mission. Sure, you can throw on a pack and head out alone with your thoughts (and maybe your favorite podcast). But when you bring other people into it, the benefits multiply.

- **Local ruck groups.** Search online or in your area—there are communities dedicated to rucking that welcome all ages and fitness levels.

- **Friends and family.** Invite your spouse, your neighbor, or your dog (okay, the dog doesn't carry weight, but they'll still love it).

- **Charity rucks.** Many organizations host rucking events to raise money for causes. You'll get fitter and make a difference.

Community adds accountability, support, and a sense f fun. It's harder to quit when someone's waiting for you at the trailhead with their own pack.

Your Next Steps (Turning Rucking Into a Lifestyle)

At this point, you know what rucking is, why it works, and how to do it safely. You've got beginner and advanced plans. You've got strategies to avoid boredom, break through plateaus, and keep moving forward. So what's next?

Here's the simple roadmap:

1. **Commit.** Pick your days, grab your pack, and make rucking part of your weekly routine.

2. **Challenge yourself.** After the 12-week plans, set bigger goals: a 10K ruck, an all-day hike, or a charity event.

3. **Stay flexible.** Life changes, schedules change, and bodies change. The beauty of rucking is that you can always adjust—lighter, shorter, slower, or heavier, longer, faster.

4. **Vacations!** One of the best ways I have found to stay motivated it to plan a vacation around a rucking event. Take a look at the Goruck website, www.goruck.com, as not only do they have a ton of knowledge and gear, but they have a lot of links to rucking events all over the Country! Not only is your vacation plan a great motivator to train, but then you'll get to meet a lot of great people and explore a new city. Ruck yeah!

Rucking isn't just exercise. It's a tool for living well. It's proof that staying strong, lean, and capable after 50 isn't a pipe dream—it's a backpack and a pair of shoes away.

The Bottom Line

Aging doesn't mean fading away. It means leaning into what works, cutting the fluff, and focusing on the simple things that pay the biggest dividends. Rucking is one of those things.

It's not flashy. It's not complicated. But it works—day after day, step after step. With every ruck, you're burning fat, strengthening your body, protecting your bones, sharpening your mind, and proving that your best years aren't behind you—they're the ones you're carrying forward.

So strap up, step out, and keep moving. Because life after 50 isn't about slowing down—it's about rucking up and powering through, one weighted step at a time.

Epilogue: Ruck Up and Step Forward

Here's the thing: you don't need me anymore.

You've read the science, laughed at the jokes, and maybe even looked suspiciously at your old backpack sitting in the closet. You now know the secret that most fitness magazines and social media influencers won't tell you: **fitness after 50 doesn't have to be complicated.** It doesn't require miracle supplements, celebrity trainers, or a personal sauna in your basement.

It requires...walking. With weight. Consistently.

That's it. That's the magic formula.

The beauty of rucking is that it's not a "program" with an end date. It's not something you do for 30 days and then quit. It's something you *live.* It's a tool you can carry with you (literally) for the rest of your life.

Every ruck you take is a declaration: *I'm not slowing down. I'm not giving in. I'm not fading away.*

You're telling your body, your brain, and the world that you still have plenty left in the tank—and you plan to use it.

So here's my challenge to you:

- Don't overthink it.

- Don't wait for Monday (which I was famous for).

- Don't worry if you have the "right" backpack.

Just grab a bag, throw in a little weight, and step out the door. Ten minutes today is better than an hour you "plan" to do tomorrow.

Because the first step isn't just the hardest—it's the most important. And once you take it, every step after gets easier.

Fifty, sixty, seventy, eighty—rucking doesn't care about your age. All it cares about is that you show up, strap in, and keep moving forward. And that, my friend, is exactly what healthy aging and lifelong fitness are all about.

So ruck up. Step out. And go claim the stronger, leaner, healthier life waiting for you—one weighted step at a time.

REFERENCES

Cpt, R. M. B. (2024, March 29). A beginner's guide to rucking. Verywell Fit. https://www.verywellfit.com/what-is-rucking-8619172

Huberman Lab Clips. (2025, June 20). How & why to ruck for weight loss & strength | Michael Easter & Dr. Andrew Huberman [Video]. YouTube. https://www.youtube.com/watch?v=6XQgkA_H7z4

JB Outside. (2021, December 31). Rucking 101: Start SLOW start SMALL! From beginner to advanced [Video]. YouTube. https://www.youtube.com/watch?v=Dk07AiKLSOE

Peter Attia MD. (2024, March 5). Answering frequently asked questions about rucking | Peter Attia and Jason McCarthy [Video]. YouTube. https://www.youtube.com/watch?v=NGP3L43G5so

Wild Hunt Conditioning – James Pieratt. (2024, February 9). The rucking bible: Everything you need to know about rucking [Video]. YouTube. https://www.youtube.com/watch?v=FqtcZ1jtoQk

www.ingramcontent.com/pod-product-compliance
Ingram Content Group UK Ltd.
Pitfield, Milton Keynes, MK11 3LW, UK
UKHW021345120326